TEIN SHAN PAI MARTIAL ARTS

Fundamentals And Methods Of Self-Defense: From Basics To Advanced Techniques

QIÁNG ZǏMÒ

Table of Contents

Introductory

Tien Shan Pai is an indigenous Chinese style of martial arts. Its comprehensive approach is renowned for its integration of components from numerous traditional Chinese martial arts systems. The English translation of "Tein Shan" is "Mountain of Heaven," an appellation that alludes to the philosophical and spiritual dimensions that are frequently highlighted in this martial art's practice.

Tein Shan Pai integrates strategies derived from Tai Chi Chuan, Northern Shaolin Kung Fu, and additional varieties of Chinese martial arts. Strikes, kicks, joint locks, throws, and weapon techniques are emphasized. In addition, internal energy cultivation, including qigong and meditation, is emphasized for the purposes of enhancing health, vitality, and martial efficacy.

Subsequent to its inception, it has garnered widespread recognition across the globe, particularly among martial arts practitioners in search of a holistic approach that encompasses mental fortitude, physical conditioning, and spiritual maturation.

CHAPTER ONE
The Core Tenets Of Tein Shan Pai

Tein Shan Pai encompasses a set of core tenets that guide its practice and philosophy. While specific teachings may vary slightly depending on the instructor or school, common principles include:

• **Martial Virtue (Wude)**: Emphasizes the cultivation of moral character, integrity, and ethical conduct both inside and outside of training. Practitioners are encouraged to exhibit respect, humility, patience, and compassion.

• **Physical Conditioning (Shenti Lian)**: Focuses on developing strength, flexibility, agility, endurance, and overall physical fitness through rigorous training regimens.

• **Technical Proficiency (Jiashi Gongfu)**: Stresses the mastery of martial arts techniques, including strikes, kicks, blocks, joint locks, throws, and weapon proficiency.

• **Internal Energy Cultivation (Neigong)**: Involves practices such as qigong, meditation, and breathing exercises to enhance internal energy (qi) flow, promote health, vitality, and increase martial effectiveness.

• **Adaptability and Fluidity (Shili)**: Encourages practitioners to be adaptable and flexible in their approach to combat, responding effectively to changing circumstances and opponents.

• **Unity of Mind, Body, and Spirit (Xin Shen Yi)**: Aims to harmonize mental focus, physical movement, and spiritual awareness to achieve a state of unity and balance.

• **Self-Defense and Personal Protection (Ziwei Baodian)**: Provides practical techniques for self-defense and personal protection, emphasizing the importance of avoiding conflict when possible and using force only as a last resort.

• **Continuous Learning and Improvement (Jixu Jingshen)**: Promotes a lifelong commitment to learning, self-improvement, and personal growth both in martial arts practice and in all aspects of life.

• Tein Shan Pai practitioners adhere to these fundamental principles, which promote a comprehensive approach to martial arts instruction that incorporates not only physical but also mental and spiritual growth. By engaging in consistent training and adhering to these tenets, individuals endeavor to develop not only physical prowess but also inward fortitude, self-awareness, and ethical character.

Comprehension Of Yang And Yin In Martial Arts

The notions of Yin and Yang, which originate in traditional Chinese philosophy, are pivotal in martial arts as they pertain to the comprehension of combat dynamics, strategy, and technique. The martial arts implement the principles of Yin and Yang as follows:

• Equilibrium and Harmony: Yin and Yang symbolize contrasting yet complementary energies. Practitioners of martial arts strive to attain a harmonious equilibrium between the Yang (active, assertive) and Yin (passive, submitting) facets. Harmony is promoted in movement, technique, and mentality through this equilibrium.

• Softness and Hardness: Yin is symbolic of docility and compliance, whereas Yang embodies resoluteness and confidence. Martial artists strategically employ both of these qualities. A soft, yielding technique, for instance, could potentially deflect an opponent's force, whereas a firm, assertive strike could capitalize on vulnerabilities in their defense.

• Flow and Structure: Yin is frequently associated with dynamic, fluid motions, while Yang is linked to methodical, linear processes. Efficient martial arts training amalgamates these attributes, merging dexterity and precision in order to produce power and command.

• Stability and Adaptability: Yin represents flexibility and adaptability, enabling practitioners to react effortlessly to evolving circumstances. Yang signifies grounding and stability, thereby establishing a sturdy framework for both technique and equilibrium.

• Cyclical Motion: Yin and Yang exhibit a dynamic and interdependent nature, perpetually undergoing a cyclical transition into each other. This notion is reflected in the dynamic interplay between offense and defense, motion and immobility, and action and reaction within the realm of martial arts.

• Energy and Intent Yin and Yang are also associated with energy (Qi) and intent (Yi), which are intrinsic facets of martial arts. Yin practices, such as breathing exercises and meditation, are utilized to teach practitioners how to leverage and cultivate Qi, while Yi is employed to direct and concentrate their intent during combat and training.

• The comprehension of Yin and Yang principles empowers martial artists to formulate efficacious strategies and tactics. By skillfully balancing adaptability and stability, as well as softness and rigidity, practitioners are able to capitalize on the weaknesses of their adversaries while minimizing their own risks.

In essence, the principles of Yin and Yang furnish a conceptual structure through which one can comprehend the ever-evolving interaction of forces within the realm of martial arts. Through the incorporation of these principles into their instructional regimen, professionals endeavor to attain a cohesive equilibrium among methodology, tactic, and mentality, thereby ultimately augmenting their proficiency, efficacy, and individual growth.

CHAPTER TWO
The Concept Of Qi And Its Role In Tein Shan Pai

In Tein Shan Pai, like in many other traditional Chinese martial arts, the concept of Qi (or Chi) plays a significant role. Qi is understood as the vital energy or life force that flows through all living beings and permeates the universe according to Chinese philosophy. Here's how the concept of Qi is incorporated into Tein Shan Pai:

• **Internal Energy Cultivation**: Tein Shan Pai emphasizes internal energy cultivation as a core aspect of training. Practitioners engage in various practices, including Qigong (energy cultivation exercises), meditation, and breathing techniques, to develop and enhance their Qi. These practices aim to increase energy circulation, promote physical health, and enhance martial effectiveness.

• **Harmonizing Yin and Yang**: Qi is seen as the bridge between Yin and Yang energies in the body. Through training, practitioners seek to harmonize the Yin (passive) and Yang (active) aspects of their energy, achieving a balanced state conducive to optimal performance in martial arts and daily life.

• **Power Generation**: In Tein Shan Pai, Qi is closely associated with the generation and application of power in techniques. By cultivating Qi through training and directing it with focused intent, practitioners can enhance the effectiveness of their strikes, blocks, and other techniques.

• **Vitality and Health**: Cultivating Qi is believed to promote overall vitality and well-being. Regular practice of Qigong and other internal energy exercises in Tein Shan Pai aims to boost the body's energy levels, strengthen the immune system, and enhance physical and mental resilience.

• **Mind-Body Integration**: Qi serves as a bridge between the mind and body, facilitating greater awareness, concentration, and control. Through mindfulness practices and focused breathing, practitioners learn to harness Qi to unify their mental focus, physical movement, and internal energy.

• **Self-Defense and Martial Skill**: Understanding and manipulating Qi is considered essential for mastering advanced martial arts techniques. By developing sensitivity to Qi flow within themselves and their opponents, practitioners can anticipate movements, exploit openings, and execute techniques with precision and efficiency.

Overall, in Tein Shan Pai, the concept of Qi is integrated into every aspect of training, from physical conditioning to martial technique to spiritual development. By cultivating and harnessing Qi, practitioners strive to achieve a holistic balance of mind, body, and spirit, ultimately enhancing their martial skill, health, and overall well-being.

Mental Discipline And Focus

Mental discipline and focus are essential components of martial arts training in Tein Shan Pai, as in many other traditional martial arts styles. Here's how mental discipline and focus are emphasized in Tein Shan Pai:

• **Concentration and Mindfulness**: Practitioners are encouraged to cultivate concentration and mindfulness during training. This involves focusing their attention fully on the present moment, whether performing techniques, sparring, or engaging in meditation or Qigong exercises. By maintaining a focused awareness, practitioners can improve their technique, refine their movements, and develop greater sensitivity to their own bodies and their opponents.

•	**Visualization**: Visualization techniques are often employed in Tein Shan Pai to enhance mental discipline and focus. Practitioners visualize themselves performing techniques with precision and effectiveness, imagining every detail of the movement, from footwork to hand placement to breathing. This mental rehearsal helps to reinforce muscle memory and develop a stronger mind-body connection.

• **Breath Control**: Control of the breath is a fundamental aspect of mental discipline in Tein Shan Pai. Practitioners learn to regulate their breathing during training, coordinating it with their movements to maximize efficiency and power. Breath control also helps to calm the mind, reduce stress, and maintain focus under pressure.

• **Goal Setting and Persistence**: Setting clear goals and maintaining a disciplined approach to training are essential for mental focus and progress in Tein Shan Pai. Practitioners set both short-term and long-term goals, whether mastering a particular technique, advancing to the next rank, or competing in tournaments. Through consistent practice and perseverance, they work steadily towards their objectives, building mental resilience and determination along the way.

• **Emotional Regulation**: Emotional control is another aspect of mental discipline emphasized in Tein Shan Pai. Practitioners learn to remain calm and composed, even in challenging or high-pressure situations. By managing their emotions effectively, they can make clearer decisions, adapt to changing circumstances, and maintain focus on their objectives.

• **Meditation and Mental Training**: Meditation is often incorporated into Tein Shan Pai training to cultivate mental discipline, clarity, and inner peace. Through regular meditation practice, practitioners develop greater self-awareness, emotional balance, and mental resilience, which are invaluable for maintaining focus both on and off the training mat.

Overall, mental discipline and focus are integral to the practice of Tein Shan Pai, enabling practitioners to develop greater skill, awareness, and self-mastery in their martial arts journey.

By cultivating these qualities, practitioners not only improve their martial abilities but also enhance their overall well-being and personal growth.

Fundamentals Of Tein Shan Pai

The fundamentals of Tein Shan Pai encompass a comprehensive approach to martial arts training, focusing on both physical techniques and mental development. Here are some key aspects of the fundamentals of Tein Shan Pai:

• **Stances and Footwork**: Tein Shan Pai emphasizes the importance of proper stances and footwork as the foundation of effective martial arts technique. Practitioners learn various stances, such as horse stance, bow stance, and cat stance, and how to transition smoothly between them.

Good footwork enables practitioners to maintain balance, mobility, and stability during movement and combat.

• **Strikes and Kicks**: Training in Tein Shan Pai includes a wide range of striking and kicking techniques. Practitioners learn to deliver punches, palm strikes, elbow strikes, and various types of kicks with speed, power, and precision. Emphasis is placed on correct body mechanics, alignment, and timing to maximize the effectiveness of each technique.

• **Blocks and Defensive Techniques**: Defensive skills are essential in Tein Shan Pai for protecting oneself from attacks and countering opponents' movements. Practitioners learn a variety of blocking techniques, including parries, deflects, and evasive maneuvers, as well as how to use their arms, legs, and body to intercept and neutralize incoming strikes.

• **Grappling and Joint Locks**: Tein Shan Pai incorporates grappling and joint locking techniques for close-quarters combat and self-defense. Practitioners learn how to control an opponent's limbs, manipulate their joints, and apply leverage to immobilize or subdue them. Training includes drills and partner exercises to develop sensitivity, timing, and positional awareness.

• **Throws and Takedowns**: Throws and takedowns are integral components of Tein Shan Pai's repertoire of techniques. Practitioners learn how to off-balance and unbalance opponents using leverage, momentum, and body mechanics, then execute throws and takedowns to bring them to the ground safely and efficiently.

• **Weapons Training**: Tein Shan Pai includes training with traditional Chinese weapons, such as staff, sword, spear, and broadsword. Practitioners learn weapon forms, techniques, and applications, developing proficiency in both solo and partner drills. Weapon training enhances coordination, agility, and adaptability, as well as deepening understanding of martial principles.

• **Internal Training**: Internal training methods, such as Qigong, meditation, and breathing exercises, are integral to Tein Shan Pai. These practices cultivate internal energy (Qi), promote relaxation, focus the mind, and enhance overall health and vitality. Internal training complements external martial arts techniques, fostering a holistic approach to physical and mental development.

• **Sparring and Application**: Sparring drills and controlled sparring are essential components of Tein Shan Pai training, allowing practitioners to apply and test their techniques in realistic combat situations. Sparring develops timing, distance, reflexes, and adaptability, while also building confidence and resilience under pressure.

By focusing on these fundamentals, practitioners of Tein Shan Pai develop a well-rounded skill set, encompassing striking, grappling, weapons, and internal training, as well as cultivating mental discipline, focus, and character development.

This comprehensive approach enables practitioners to become proficient martial artists capable of defending themselves effectively, promoting health and well-being, and embodying the principles of martial virtue in their daily lives.

CHAPTER THREE
Blocks And Defense Techniques

Blocks and defensive techniques are vital components of martial arts training in Tein Shan Pai. Here are some common blocks and defensive techniques employed in the style:

Basic Blocks:

• **High Block (Jiho Gyeorugi)**: Used to deflect or intercept high-line attacks such as punches or strikes aimed at the head or shoulders.

• **Middle Block (Chungyo Gyeorugi)**: Deflects or redirects attacks aimed at the midsection or torso, including punches, kicks, or strikes.

• **Low Block (Najunde Gyeorugi)**: Used to defend against low-line attacks such as kicks or strikes aimed at the legs, groin, or lower body.

Open Hand Defenses:

• **Palm Strike (Son Deung Mok Chigi)**: Utilizes the open palm to intercept or push away incoming attacks, redirecting the opponent's force.

• **Knife Hand Block (Sonkal Makgi)**: The edge of the hand is used to block or intercept strikes, providing a wider surface area for defense.

Evasive Maneuvers:

• **Slip and Roll**: Involves moving the body out of the path of an attack, often by slipping to the side or rolling under incoming strikes.

• **Duck and Cover**: Dropping the body and covering the head and vital areas with the arms to defend against high-line attacks.

Counterattacks from Defense:

• **Simultaneous Block and Strike (Hap Gyeorugi)**: Combines a defensive block with an immediate counterattack, exploiting openings created by the opponent's attack.

- **Counter Grabs and Joint Locks**: When an opponent initiates a grab or clinch, practitioners can counter with joint locks, escapes, or throws to neutralize the threat and gain control.

Parries and Redirects:

- **Outside Parry**: Redirects an incoming strike away from the practitioner's body, often followed by a counterattack.

- **Inside Parry**: Similar to the outside parry but redirects the attack inward, setting up opportunities for counters or follow-up techniques.

Clinch Defense:

• **Clinch Breaks**: Techniques to escape or break free from an opponent's clinch, including strikes, leverage, and footwork to create distance.

• **Clinch Defense and Counters**: Utilizes techniques such as arm drags, hip throws, or sweeps to defend against and counter opponents attempting to engage in close-quarters combat.

These are just a few examples of the blocks and defensive techniques employed in Tein Shan Pai. Mastery of these techniques requires practice, timing, and sensitivity to the opponent's movements, enabling practitioners to effectively defend themselves while maintaining control and composure in combat situations.

Forms And Kata

Forms, also known as "kata" in Japanese martial arts, are prearranged sequences of movements that are practiced as a way to develop technique, strength, speed, balance, and focus in martial arts.

In Tein Shan Pai, practitioners learn various forms that encompass a wide range of techniques and principles. These forms are typically performed solo, though some may involve partner drills or applications.

Here are some common forms practiced in Tein Shan Pai:

• **Tiger Form (Houquan)**: The Tiger form emphasizes powerful, explosive movements reminiscent of the tiger's strength and agility. It typically includes strong strikes, low stances, and dynamic footwork.

• **Crane Form (Hequan)**: The Crane form emphasizes grace, balance, and fluidity, mimicking the movements of the crane. It often includes sweeping, circular movements, precise strikes, and evasive footwork.

• **Dragon Form (Longquan)**: The Dragon form focuses on cultivating internal energy, flexibility, and control.

It incorporates flowing, spiraling movements, dynamic shifts in speed and direction, and techniques that harness the dragon's mythical power.

• **Snake Form (Shequan)**: The Snake form emphasizes speed, precision, and agility, drawing inspiration from the snake's stealth and striking ability. It includes rapid strikes, intricate hand techniques, and fluid, sinuous movements.

• **Five-Animal Form (Wu Xing Quan)**: The Five-Animal form integrates movements inspired by the characteristics of various animals, including tiger, crane, dragon, snake, and leopard. It provides a comprehensive training regimen that develops different aspects of martial skill and energy cultivation.

• **Weapon Forms**: In addition to empty-hand forms, Tein Shan Pai includes forms for various traditional Chinese weapons, such as staff, sword, spear, and broadsword. Weapon forms incorporate techniques specific to each weapon, as well as principles of timing, distance, and strategy.

• **Self-Defense Applications**: Some forms in Tein Shan Pai include practical self-defense applications, where practitioners demonstrate how techniques from the form can be used in real-life combat situations. These applications help practitioners understand the practical relevance of the movements and develop their ability to apply them effectively.

• **Advanced Forms and Specialized Training**: As practitioners progress in their training, they may learn more advanced forms that challenge their skills and deepen their understanding of martial principles. Specialized forms may focus on specific aspects of training, such as internal energy cultivation, sparring, or weapon techniques.

Forms practice in Tein Shan Pai serves multiple purposes, including physical conditioning, technical proficiency, mental focus, and aesthetic expression.

Through diligent practice of forms, practitioners develop a deeper understanding of martial arts principles, enhance their overall skill level, and cultivate a sense of discipline, concentration, and mastery in their practice.

CHAPTER FOUR
Application Of Forms In Combat

In Tein Shan Pai, as in many other martial arts styles, the application of forms in combat is a crucial aspect of training. While forms practice primarily focuses on developing technique, balance, coordination, and other fundamental skills, practitioners also learn to apply the movements and principles learned in forms to real-life self-defense situations. Here's how forms are applied in combat within the context of Tein Shan Pai:

• **Technique Familiarization**: Forms practice allows practitioners to become familiar with a wide range of techniques, including strikes, blocks, kicks, joint locks, throws, and combinations thereof. Through repetition and refinement of form movements, practitioners develop muscle memory and fluidity in executing techniques, which can be applied spontaneously in combat situations.

• **Timing and Distance**: Forms training helps practitioners understand the appropriate timing and distance for executing techniques effectively. By practicing the movements within the context of a form, practitioners learn to judge the timing of attacks and defenses, as well as how to close or maintain distance with opponents to maximize the effectiveness of their techniques.

• **Combination Techniques**: Many forms in Tein Shan Pai involve sequences of movements that flow seamlessly from one technique to another. Practitioners learn to link these movements together into effective combinations that can be used in combat. By practicing forms with a focus on fluid transitions and timing, practitioners develop the ability to chain techniques together in response to changing situations in combat.

• **Adaptability and Creativity**: While forms provide a structured framework for training, practitioners also learn to adapt and improvise based on the specific circumstances of a combat encounter. Through application drills and sparring, practitioners learn to apply the principles and techniques learned in forms in dynamic, unpredictable situations, developing the ability to respond flexibly and creatively to different opponents and scenarios.

• **Visualization and Mental Training**: Forms practice encourages practitioners to visualize themselves in combat situations, imagining opponents attacking from various angles and distances. This mental training helps practitioners develop strategic thinking, spatial awareness, and tactical decision-making skills, which are essential for effective combat application.

• **Partner Drills and Application Training**: In addition to solo forms practice, Tein Shan Pai includes partner drills and application training exercises where practitioners practice applying techniques from forms in controlled, cooperative settings. These drills allow practitioners to refine their timing, accuracy, and sensitivity to their opponent's movements, preparing them for live sparring and real-world self-defense scenarios.

Overall, the application of forms in combat within Tein Shan Pai is a dynamic and multifaceted process that involves integrating the techniques, principles, and mental training developed through forms practice into practical self-defense skills. Through diligent training and application, practitioners learn to adapt and respond effectively to the challenges of combat, ultimately enhancing their martial proficiency and readiness for real-world encounters.

Techniques And Drills For Weapon Handling

In Tein Shan Pai, weapon handling is an essential component of training, encompassing a wide range of techniques and drills designed to develop proficiency with traditional Chinese weapons. Here are some common techniques and drills for weapon handling in Tein Shan Pai:

• **Basic Grips and Stances**: Practitioners begin by learning the proper grips and stances for each weapon. This includes understanding how to hold the weapon securely and comfortably, as well as adopting appropriate stances that provide stability, mobility, and balance.

• **Solo Forms Practice**: Weapon forms, or "taolu," are prearranged sequences of movements that practitioners perform solo to develop technique, coordination, and fluidity with the weapon. Each weapon has its own set of forms that incorporate strikes, blocks, footwork, and other techniques specific to that weapon.

• **Partner Drills and Applications**: Partner drills and applications involve practicing techniques with a training partner, simulating various combat scenarios and responses. These drills may include offensive and defensive techniques, counters, and combinations, allowing practitioners to refine their timing, distance, and accuracy in applying techniques with the weapon.

• **Sparring with Weapons**: Weapon sparring involves engaging in controlled, simulated combat with a training partner using padded or blunted weapons. Practitioners practice applying techniques learned in forms and drills in a dynamic, live environment, testing their skills, reactions, and adaptability under pressure.

• **Target Practice**: Practicing striking and thrusting techniques on targets such as pads, dummies, or wooden targets helps practitioners develop power, accuracy, and precision with the weapon. Target practice also reinforces proper technique and body mechanics, allowing practitioners to refine their striking skills.

• **Disarming Techniques**: Learning how to disarm opponents wielding weapons is an important aspect of weapon training in Tein Shan Pai.

Practitioners practice techniques for disarming opponents safely and effectively, including controlling the weapon, applying joint locks, and using leverage to neutralize threats.

• **Forms with Multiple Opponents**: Some weapon forms in Tein Shan Pai simulate scenarios where practitioners must defend against multiple attackers. These forms teach practitioners how to move, position themselves, and use the weapon strategically to overcome multiple opponents while minimizing exposure to danger.

• **Weapon Spinning and Flourishes**: Weapon spinning and flourishes are advanced techniques that add flair and fluidity to weapon handling.

Practitioners learn to manipulate the weapon with precision and control, performing intricate spinning, flipping, and twirling movements that demonstrate mastery and dexterity with the weapon.

Overall, weapon handling in Tein Shan Pai encompasses a combination of solo practice, partner drills, sparring, and specialized techniques designed to develop skill, confidence, and effectiveness with traditional Chinese weapons. Through diligent training and practice, practitioners learn to wield weapons with precision, power, and grace, embodying the principles of martial virtue and discipline in their martial arts journey.

CHAPTER FIVE
Combat Applications Of Weapons

In Tein Shan Pai, like in many traditional martial arts styles, weapons are considered extensions of the practitioner's body and are taught with a focus on practical combat applications. Here are some common combat applications of weapons in Tein Shan Pai:

• **Striking Techniques**: Weapons such as staffs, swords, and spears are used to deliver powerful strikes to an opponent. Practitioners learn various striking techniques, including thrusts, slashes, sweeps, and chops, aimed at vulnerable targets such as vital areas, joints, and limbs.

• **Blocking and Parrying**: Weapons can be used defensively to block or parry incoming attacks from opponents. Practitioners learn how to intercept strikes with their weapon, deflecting or redirecting the force of the attack while maintaining their own balance and stability.

• **Disarming and Control**: Weapons training in Tein Shan Pai includes techniques for disarming opponents wielding weapons, as well as methods for controlling and neutralizing threats. Practitioners learn joint locks, pressure points, and leverage techniques to disarm opponents safely and effectively, minimizing the risk of injury.

• **Close-Quarters Combat**: In close-quarters combat, weapons such as knives or short staffs can be used to strike, stab, or incapacitate opponents at close range. Practitioners learn techniques for quick, decisive action in confined spaces, utilizing the weapon's reach and versatility to gain the upper hand in combat.

• **Multiple Opponents**: Weapons can be effective tools for defending against multiple attackers. Practitioners learn how to use their weapon to create space, control the engagement, and neutralize threats from multiple directions, minimizing their exposure to danger and maximizing their chances of survival.

• **Feinting and Deception**: Weapons can be used to feint or deceive opponents, creating openings for counterattacks or escapes. Practitioners learn how to manipulate their weapon with precision and timing, luring opponents into committing to a particular attack before exploiting weaknesses in their defense.

• **Environmental Adaptation**: Weapons training in Tein Shan Pai emphasizes adaptability and resourcefulness in combat. Practitioners learn to assess their surroundings and use objects in the environment to their advantage, incorporating improvised weapons or obstacles into their strategy as needed.

- **Strategy and Tactics**: Weapons training goes beyond mere technique, encompassing strategic thinking and tactical awareness in combat. Practitioners learn how to assess opponents, anticipate their movements, and formulate effective strategies for overcoming them, whether through direct confrontation, evasion, or subterfuge.

Overall, combat applications of weapons in Tein Shan Pai emphasize practicality, efficiency, and adaptability, preparing practitioners to defend themselves effectively in a variety of real-world situations. Through diligent training and practice, practitioners develop the skills, confidence, and mindset necessary to wield weapons with skill and precision, embodying the principles of martial virtue and discipline in their martial arts journey.

Sparring And Combat Techniques

Sparring and combat techniques in Tein Shan Pai involve the application of martial arts principles in dynamic, live situations. Here are some common sparring and combat techniques used in the style:

• **Footwork and Movement**: Effective footwork is essential for maintaining proper distance, angle, and positioning during sparring. Practitioners use footwork techniques such as shuffling, pivoting, circling, and angling to control the engagement, create openings, and evade opponents' attacks.

• **Striking Techniques**: Striking techniques are fundamental in sparring and combat. Practitioners use punches, palm strikes, elbow strikes, and kicks to deliver powerful, accurate blows to opponents. Emphasis is placed on proper technique, timing, and target selection to maximize effectiveness while minimizing exposure to counterattacks.

• **Blocking and Defense**: Blocking and defensive techniques are crucial for protecting oneself from opponents' attacks during sparring. Practitioners use techniques such as high blocks, low blocks, parries, and evasive maneuvers to intercept or deflect incoming strikes, maintaining a strong defense while seeking opportunities to counterattack.

• **Counterattacks**: Counterattacking is an essential aspect of sparring and combat in Tein Shan Pai. Practitioners learn to capitalize on openings created by opponents' attacks, responding with swift, decisive counterattacks. This may involve countering strikes with strikes, blocking and returning fire, or using leverage and positioning to gain the advantage.

• **Clinch Fighting**: Clinch fighting occurs when practitioners engage in close-quarters combat, grappling for control or attempting takedowns.

Practitioners use techniques such as clinch breaks, arm drags, sweeps, and throws to gain leverage and control over opponents, either to neutralize their attacks or set up follow-up techniques.

• **Takedowns and Throws**: Takedowns and throws are effective techniques for controlling opponents and dictating the pace of a sparring or combat encounter. Practitioners use techniques such as hip throws, shoulder throws, and leg sweeps to off-balance opponents and bring them to the ground, gaining a dominant position from which to follow up with strikes or submissions.

- **Submission Techniques**: Submission techniques involve applying joint locks, chokes, or other holds to force opponents to submit or yield. While sparring is typically non-contact and does not involve submissions, practitioners may practice submission techniques in controlled drilling or in more advanced training settings.

- **Strategy and Tactics**: Sparring and combat in Tein Shan Pai require strategic thinking and tactical awareness. Practitioners learn to assess opponents, adapt their tactics, and exploit weaknesses in their defense. This may involve feinting, baiting, or setting traps to lure opponents into committing to attacks before countering with their own techniques.

Overall, sparring and combat techniques in Tein Shan Pai encompass a diverse range of skills, including striking, blocking, grappling, and strategy. Through diligent training and practice, practitioners develop the proficiency, confidence, and adaptability necessary to navigate dynamic combat situations effectively, embodying the principles of martial virtue and discipline in their martial arts journey.

CHAPTER SIX
Conditioning And Training Methods'

Conditioning and training methods in Tein Shan Pai are designed to develop physical fitness, martial skills, mental discipline, and internal energy cultivation. Here are some common conditioning and training methods used in the style:

• **Basic Physical Conditioning**: Tein Shan Pai training includes exercises to develop strength, endurance, flexibility, and cardiovascular fitness. This may include bodyweight exercises such as push-ups, sit-ups, squats, lunges, and burpees, as well as calisthenics, plyometrics, and cardiovascular workouts such as running or jump rope.

• **Martial Arts Techniques Practice**: Practitioners spend time refining their martial arts techniques through repetition, partner drills, and shadowboxing. This includes practicing strikes, blocks, kicks, joint locks, throws, and other techniques with a focus on proper form, timing, and application.

• **Forms Practice (Taolu)**: Forms practice involves performing choreographed sequences of movements that incorporate various martial arts techniques. Forms practice helps develop muscle memory, coordination, balance, and fluidity in movement, as well as mental focus and discipline.

- **Sparring and Partner Drills**: Sparring and partner drills allow practitioners to apply their techniques in dynamic, live situations. This helps develop timing, distance, accuracy, and adaptability in combat, as well as enhancing tactical awareness, strategy, and decision-making under pressure.

- **Weapon Training**: Weapon training includes practicing techniques with traditional Chinese weapons such as staff, sword, spear, and broadsword. This involves learning forms, solo drills, partner drills, and sparring with weapons, developing proficiency, coordination, and adaptability in weapon handling.

• **Qigong and Internal Training**: Qigong and internal training methods are integral to Tein Shan Pai, emphasizing energy cultivation, relaxation, and mental focus. This may include practicing breathing exercises, meditation, visualization, and mindfulness techniques to enhance physical and mental well-being, as well as martial effectiveness.

• **Strength and Conditioning Equipment**: Tein Shan Pai training may incorporate the use of strength and conditioning equipment such as kettlebells, resistance bands, medicine balls, and agility ladders to enhance functional strength, power, speed, and agility.

• **Cross-Training**: Cross-training in complementary disciplines such as yoga, tai chi, gymnastics, or weightlifting may be incorporated into Tein Shan Pai training to enhance overall physical fitness, mobility, and body awareness.

• **Rest and Recovery**: Adequate rest and recovery are essential aspects of Tein Shan Pai training to prevent overtraining, reduce the risk of injury, and promote physical and mental rejuvenation. Practitioners are encouraged to listen to their bodies, get sufficient sleep, and incorporate rest days into their training regimen.

In its entirety, Tein Shan Pai incorporates a wide range of conditioning and training techniques that encompass the physical, mental, and spiritual dimensions of the martial arts discipline.

By engaging in rigorous training and maintaining a consistent practice of these techniques, individuals cultivate the aptitudes, qualities, and mentality that are essential for advancing in their pursuit of martial arts and attaining their objectives.

Implementing Tein Shan Pai In Everyday Life

The incorporation of Tein Shan Pai into one's daily life transcends mere physical exertion; it entails the complete embodiment of martial arts principles and values across all facets of existence. Tein Shan Pai can be implemented in the following methods into one's daily life:

• Cultivate mindfulness and awareness by directing your attention towards your thoughts, emotions, and actions during your daily activities. Utilize the concentration and focus that martial arts training has fostered to accomplish tasks at home, in the workplace, or in the classroom.

• Physical Health and Fitness: Sustain a consistent exercise regimen to preserve your physical fitness. Incorporate daily components of Tein Shan Pai training into your regimen, including cardiovascular exercise, strength training, and stretching, in order to enhance your overall health.

• Ethical Conduct and Integrity: In all your engagements with others, adhere to the principles of martial virtue, which comprise integrity, compassion, humility, and respect. Consider yourself an exemplar of positivity and conduct others with courtesy, decency, and esteem.

• The Importance of Self-Control and Discipline: Incorporate self-control and discipline into every aspect of your life by establishing objectives, managing your time efficiently, and resisting temptation and diversion. In order to surmount obstacles and attain triumph, employ the tenacity and resolve that are nurtured via martial arts practice.

• Conflict Resolution and Communication: Employ martial arts principles to assertively and amicably resolve conflicts in social interactions, professional contexts, and personal relationships. Foster comprehension and unity by employing active listening, empathy, and effective communication techniques.

• Lifelong Learning and Development: Adopt an attitude of perpetual learning and development, actively pursuing opportunities to broaden your horizons, expertise, and understanding. By incorporating martial arts principles—namely adaptability, resilience, and open-mindedness—into one's life and professional development, one can effectively navigate the challenges that arise along the way.

• Community Engagement and Service: Contribute to the betterment of others and give back to your community by participating in volunteer initiatives, mentoring programs, or charitable endeavors. Employ your expertise and understanding in martial arts to motivate and enable individuals, thereby cultivating an atmosphere of cohesion, advocacy, and societal accountability.

• Commit to the Practice of Self-Reflection and Inner Growth: Schedule periods for introspection, self-reflection, and personal development. Engage in mindfulness practices such as journaling, meditation, or other methods to foster self-awareness, emotional resilience, and spiritual development.

By incorporating these aspects of Tein Shan Pai into their everyday routines, practitioners can foster a holistic approach to personal development, which includes the promotion of physical health, mental well-being, and moral integrity in both themselves and others, in addition to the enhancement of their martial arts prowess.

Summary

Tein Shan Pai is an all-encompassing system comprising physical training, mental discipline, and spiritual development; it is not merely a style of martial arts. Tein Shan Pai, which is based on the philosophy and principles of traditional Chinese martial arts, places significant emphasis on the development of martial virtue, integrity, and self-mastery across all spheres of existence.

By engaging in consistent and methodical application of forms, techniques, sparring, and conditioning routines, practitioners enhance their physical fitness, combat prowess, and technical expertise. Practitioners of Tein Shan Pai, nevertheless, gain knowledge and insight that transcend the confines of the dojo, as they discover ways to incorporate the dojo's tenets and values into their everyday existence.

Pupils of Tein Shan Pai aspire to develop not only martial prowess but also virtuous character, thereby making constructive contributions to their localities and society at large, through the embodiment of virtues including mindfulness, respect, self-discipline, and compassion.

Tein Shan Pai's voyage culminates in a process of self-exploration, individual development, and ongoing progress. Beyond the realm of physical training, the principles and practices of Tein Shan Pai offer a comprehensive structure for fostering mental, spiritual, and physical wellness. These practices and principles enable practitioners to confront the trials and tribulations of existence with composure, fortitude, and intrinsic fortitude.

THE END